A PILOT'S GUIDE TO BEATING JET LAG FOR GOOD

Tips For Staying Fully
Refreshed When You Travel

S PRICE

© **Copyright (2019) by S Price. All rights reserved.**

It is not legal to reproduce, duplicate, or transmit any part of this document in either electronic means or printed format. The recording of this publication is strictly prohibited.

S Price

Authors Disclaimer

This book is based solely on the authors' own experience, research, beliefs, and opinions. It is not intended to treat, diagnose, or prevent any illness or condition you may suffer from.

The information contained within this book is not to be a substitute for advice from a registered physician or any other health care professional.

This is only a guide and therefore readers should conduct their own research and consult with their own preferred medical practitioner before making any decisions which may concern their health. That being said, please enjoy.

CONTENTS

- Introduction
- What Is Jet lag?
- How To Sleep Anywhere!
- Shaping Your Sleep
- Tips And Tricks
- Taking Your Children Away
- Overcoming The Dreaded Sleep Deficit
- The Coffee Conundrum
- The Best Ideas When In Your Seat
- Unleashing Your Inner Hypochondriac
- The Quickest Way To Wake Up Alert
- Food And Health Tips
- Highly Effective Habits
- My Struggle As A Commercial Pilot
- The Only Way Is Up!
- What Did You Think?
- Notes

INTRODUCTION

Travelling the world is a bucket list item for most people. Whether it's to explore the marvels of the seven wonders of the world, to witness the magic of the northern lights, or to experience the sheer magnitude of the Amazon rainforest. Nothing can beat the sense of freedom that modern air travel can offer; Yet all of these everlasting memories can be so easily tarnished by the effects of jet lag. We all know that feeling when you're so tired you simply don't know whether you're in New York or the New year!

Jet lag comes in many shapes and sizes and has the potential to ruin the foundations of any trip, without any warning. This book will give you a better understanding of the habits and practices that you can easily adopt to ensure you get the best out of all of your flying adventures.

As a commercial pilot, I have faced many of these issues and have known many people who persevered to the sweet-bitter end. I have tried to collate all of these ideas in one, easy-to-read book. It's a short book and definitely one to reread before your next holiday.

Many people are still struggling with jet lag issues. This leads to a lot of wasted time when abroad, lots of missed opportunities, and a lot of disappointment. If you've ever been on a long flight, you'll know the feeling you have the few days after landing. All you want to do is go to sleep, recover from the trip, lounge around, and waste time in the hotel.

This book will teach you all of the fundamentals to utilise and build upon. It provides secret insights into the aviation industry to allow you to feel fully recovered. These tips and tricks are the best way to enjoy your holiday and ensure your health for years to come. Flights nowadays are ultimately unhealthy, and we need a solution to allow us to continue with our adventures in the best way possible.

This book has helped many people to feel healthier and happier while travelling. I collected this information over the course of my career and have finally put pen to paper and I hope to help many. As a pilot I needed to make sure I was in top form at all times; I make sure to use all of the tricks contained in my book before I go flying so I feel fully refreshed at all times. Being a commercial pilot is a most rewarding career; however, tiredness and fatigue can set in if you don't take preventative measures quickly. I gained experience fairly rapidly and now, thankfully, I have some methods to avoid going down the wrong path.

Now make sure you read this book before you next go on your holidays; it's not too late. It's a quick read that is to the point. It is a one-stop-shop for all your travelling needs. I added a few pages for notes at the back to help you keep track of the places you visit and how you feel. Use the notes pages as an aide-memoire to guide you into the habits you should be keeping before, during, and after your flight—habits that will help you feel healthy.

Good luck with all your adventures, and I wish you all the best while eliminating jet lag from your life once and for all.

WHAT IS JET LAG?

Awful. That's pretty much all you need to know.

But seriously it's not a nice thing to go through. Jet lag is your body adjusting to the time difference of flights. Through evolution, we were never designed to travel the ways in which we do today. Going through multiple time zones and seeing the sun rise/set on numerous occasions on the same day was simply not possible. No horse in the world could have been that quick.

Jet lag occurs when a person's sleep-wake cycle is disturbed. It can cause some really detrimental side effects, which are sure to ruin your holiday. It can make you drowsy, irritable, lethargic, and generally disoriented. The older a person is, the more severe the effects will be. Children usually recover amazingly well to most things, including jet lag. They may be up and ready to go after a long flight, whereas most adults will want to curl into a tiny ball on the hotel bed.

A key influence on your internal clock is sunlight. It controls and manages your melatonin, a hormone that helps synchronise the cells throughout your body. At night, the hypothalamus tells the pineal gland, a small gland in your brain, to release melatonin. During daytime hours the opposite occurs and you'll feel awake. During a flight, the sun can rise and set in one sitting. This can completely throw off your internal body clock and it will send your body into a complete meltdown. You may struggle to get to sleep at the correct time or feel completely lethargic when trying to wake up in the morning.

Medicines simply won't help you when it comes to jet lag. Herbal remedied, such as teas, may help alleviate the symptoms and will certainly help if you're struggling to get to sleep but ultimately you will still end up feeling groggy for at least a few days after flying.

Now, some of you bright sparks out there will be thinking of melatonin supplements. Unfortunately, I can't suggest them for both personal reasons, i.e. tried them and they might as well have been jelly beans; and also, medical reasons, as there is little to no proof that they work. Sorry but no shortcuts here.

Nowadays life's a lot faster paced and you can race around the world pretty darn easily. Jet lag can be a real drag on a person's travels and can also bring a great deal of stress, which has a massively detrimental effect on your health. I'll touch on this later. People today are feeling a lot worse off, and I'm here to help out with this problem as much as I can.

Fortunately, whilst you most likely won't be able to eliminate jet lag from your life altogether, there are more than a few strategies which you can try to greatly lessen the effects for yourself and your family.

HOW TO SLEEP ANYWHERE!

Starting off, there are many ways people swear will help you sleep. If you've found something that works, then great! If, on the other hand, like me, you struggle to get to sleep, then this little chapter is for you. I've been told a few different ways; I won't dive into all of them, but I'll try my best to describe the very best way I've found most helpful throughout my career.

The first thing to do if you're trying to get to sleep at the end of the day is to put down the gadgets. Blue light keeps your brain active and awake. A red light, on the other hand, is quite useful for us pilots as it maintains night vision and doesn't disrupt your natural sleep cycle too much. If you notice, that's why newer phones are incorporating a night shift to a redder colour. If, however, you can't do that and you're trying to fall asleep at the drop of a hat, you probably won't have the luxury of ditching all your tech gadgets. These techniques may take a tad longer to kick in.

I have found that visualizing something specific is the ultimate way to get to sleep. Aural thoughts, (your inner voice) keep you wide awake and you start thinking more and more. You question the things you say inside your head and you can always find yourself going on a weird tangent. Try to imagine a place, thing, or a sequence of actions. For example, driving your car to work. Imagine the route and the signs along the way. Don't say the route but imagine actually doing it. I imagine the stages of setting up on the airbus, actually pretty boring and tedious, but that's kind of the point. Anytime your mind begins to *say* something and you hear your inner voice, just try to imagine something visuallly instead. Imagine an orange rolling down the hill, a go-cart, biscuit tin, whatever you want. Just try to focus on the image, try to visualise it in all its glory and trust me, you'll be out like a light!

After studying psychology, I don't claim to be an expert, but this is what I believe is happening. The idea behind all of this is the age-old anecdote of doing two things at once. You will find that multitasking is actually pretty easy, as long as you don't try using the same areas of the brain. If you had to pat your head and say "hello" this would be easy; however, if you had to pat your head and rub your stomach that's not as easily done. This is because you'd be doing an aural task and a motor task with the first example and doing two motor tasks on the second example. It's the same with sleep; just limit the aural tasks going on in your head and you will fall asleep very easily by thinking of actions instead.

Avoid drinks containing caffeine. It's interesting to note that caffeine activates the exact same receptors in the brain as cocaine. Caffeine alters your brain chemistry which in turn speeds up your neural activity. This means that when you're trying to get to sleep, your brain is more active than ever. Caffeine can have the exact same withdrawal symptoms as cocaine as well; headaches, nausea, and dependancy.. maybe time to wean off coffee? Don't fear caffeine addicts, I'll be talking more about coffee in an upcoming chapter.

Try to avoid getting stressed out, and try some relaxation techniques. There are some great podcasts too which help you fall asleep. I've personally tried audiobooks, relaxing music playlists, and meditation apps. Meditation can aid in getting you into a very relaxed state and is definitely worth a try! These can be a big help to an even greater number of people.

I have found breathing techniques to be a Godsend. The one I've found most useful is to first exhale completely through your mouth while lying down quietly. Then inhale through your nose for around 4 seconds. Hold your breath for the count of 7 seconds. Then exhale for the count of 8 seconds. It's a quick and easy thing to try while you're in bed. It helps to relax your entire body before falling to sleep.

If someone says they fell asleep reading your book, you'd be pretty peeved. I, however, will take it as a compliment if you fall asleep reading mine, so feel free to let your mind wander and drift off into that beautiful, blissful sleep.

SHAPING YOUR SLEEP

There are three main categories of sleep. These are Rapid Eye Movement (REM), Light Sleep, and Deep Sleep. The amount of sleep you need varies from person to person, but normally around 7-9 hours is enough. In a normal bedtime routine, you'll probably be getting enough of each, but on a flight, you definitely won't be. It's your job, therefore, to shape what sleep you are getting to maximise the effects, and I'm here to help!

Generally, women need more sleep than men by around 20 minutes per night; however, this varies from person to person. Making sure that you know roughly how much sleep you need is a great place to start and is helpful in making sure you feel okay when starting your journey across the seas.

Sun light has such a big impact on how well you will sleep that night. Try to get some daily sunlight exposure or if you struggle sleeping at home, maybe invest in an artificial bright-light devices. They really can help to sleep better at night time.

Meal times on the aeroplane, when flying

across multiple time zones, can be confusing, to say the least. As mentioned before, make sure to pay attention to the crew and if they're eating when you are. It's okay to ask to postpone your meal if it seems a little too early or too late, failing that, keep it on the tray table you have in front of you. You'll want to avoid heavy meals before trying to get to sleep and instead, opt for the lite-bite snack. Meals play a huge role in how your body will adapt and feel throughout the day. Never underestimate the power of your stomach when it comes to feeling healthy and refreshed on an aeroplane.

Your heart rate is actually a great indicator of your sleep. If you have any gadgets which track your heart rate, they are very useful. The resting heart rate for adults is 40-100 beats per minute. It is good to have a slightly lower heart rate when asleep than when awake. This rate will depend upon the individual, so you would have to look at this over time.

Your body temperature will change all the time, not only throughout the day but also during the night. It's an important factor in how easily you fall to sleep and how refreshed you'll feel. As you start to fall to sleep, your body temperature will drop. Make sure you have a room slightly cooler than you would normally. You can always curl up in the duvet for a bit of warmth if you start to freeze.

Sleep pressure is when you reach the end of a day and you find it harder and harder to stay awake. It's your body's natural way of letting you know that it's time to head to bed. Adenosine is yet another chemical that is constantly building up in our bodies and acts alongside serotonin. During wakeful hours, adenosine gradually builds up in areas of our brains that are important for maintaining our aroused state. Adenosine slows down the activity and firing of neurons. With higher and higher concentrations this will then cause sleepiness and sleep pressure. Naps, throughout the day, will reduce the levels of adenosine a little, whereas a restful night of sleep will reduce the amount significantly. It's going to be useful to time your sleep patterns to fit in with your flight schedule and try to pre-plan when naps will be needed and when you'll need to fight the urge, sleep pressure, and stay awake to get a fully recovering sleep instead.

A Pilot's Guide To Beating Jet Lag For Good

TIPS AND TRICKS

Buy a flight pillow. Those things are a lifesaver. Not really the comfiest but a lot better than leaning your head on the side of a noisy plane, that's for sure! Sleep is the main goal while on any flight. Those pillows are inexpensive compared to the cost of your holiday. Time is money while abroad so £10 for a pillow certainly won't break the bank but missing a couple of days holiday feeling miserable will cost you dearly.

Invest some money in good earplugs. Cheap ones are fine for short flights, usually the little spongy ones. On long flights, earplugs are especially useful. The noise on a plane is loud; you just don't notice that much because you get used to it. After a long flight, your ears will definitely be ringing. I've pulled out a little app on my phone in the flight deck multiple times and honestly, it registers around the same noise levels as power tools or an alarm clock. I wouldn't like an alarm clock strapped to my ear for 16 hours. Not a good way to live.

When the crew onboard lower the lights, take

that as a sign to go to sleep. Take their actions as gospel and you shouldn't go too far wrong. If they serve you food, eat it. If they serve you drinks, drink it. They know the rules for the long haul and they do it a lot, so trust me and the crew!

Now this one won't be the most pleasant to think about, I'll be honest. But if you've ever been through this you'll know what I'm talking about. Diarrhea. Not enjoyable that's for sure and even less so when you are stuck in a tube hurtling along at 500 miles an hour having to step over your fellow passengers 15 times so you can go to the tiny toilet. I recommend you always travel with anti-diarrhea tablets in your bag.

Vaseline is a great purchase to get you through those long flights. Rather odd purchase and you're probably wondering what to do with it . . . not what you're thinking probably! What you want to do is lightly spread it just on the inside of your nose. It's great for keeping your airways clear and stops it from drying out. It keeps germs at bay, aiding your body, and also helps to keep you feeling refreshed. It may seem a tad odd, so I'd go to the bathroom to apply it and make it a small amount.

Cold showers are absolutely fantastic. Not only do they wake you up pretty much instantly, but they've been shown to aid your body naturally as well. They will increase your metabolism; they are great for burning off that extra bit of chocolate you ate last night, and they increase the number of white blood cells in your body which helps to fight disease. Your overall blood flow will increase and this means better circulation all around. Now I must admit it's not the most fun in the beginning. I try to gradually decrease the temperature of the shower over a weekly timeframe.

Make sure to take a black pen with you when you travel. You'd be amazed at how useful it can be, especially when you have some last-minute forms to sign, say, to bring in antihistamines into the country. I mention 'black', I once went to New Zealand and had to wait 2 hours for a new form on the ground at security because it was filled in red ink. Definitely not how I wanted to spend the start of my holiday, that's for sure.

Cables, gadgets, and chargers. You have been warned. Your gadgets are life-savers for passing the time and also helping get through the airport with ease. So many airlines nowadays have apps you can download for boarding passes, gate information, and reports on any delays. You'll want to buy a decent battery pack to keep everything charged and ready for action. If you're using them to entertain your children, all of your gadgets will definitely be flat by the time it comes to board the aeroplane.

TAKING YOUR CHILDREN AWAY

Children can often find it difficult whilst going away on holiday. From the early morning start, all the way through security and then when on the plane. It really can be an uphill struggle. First, and foremost, you'll be wanting some entertainment. Make sure to pack those gadgets, books, and games. Keeping the wait time, which you'll inevitably have, to a minimum amount of hassle.

The issues at security you'll face can be resolved with a little pre-planning. Children seem to hoard stuff everywhere. In all of their pockets you'll find loads of junk, which usually send the metal detector into over-drive. I was once behind a kid who proceeded to pull out around 15 assorted springs from his pocket, after being thwarted by the metal detector. One of those springs worked wonders to fix my wheely bag, I digress.

The night before getting ready, go through with your children what will be happening at the security gates. Make it into a game to put all their objects into the little plastic bags as quickly as possible and make sure to check they haven't forgotten anything which may set off those, wonderfully sensitive, machines they have at security.

Waiting in the terminal is a nightmare for anyone - so when you're young, even worse. There are some great viewing platforms in most terminals to go and do a bit of plane spotting, just ask a staff member. Make sure to grab a few bottles of water whilst you're in the terminal as well, both you and your kids will be dehydrated after waiting for the flight.

Well, that's it. You're on the plane. No more worries. Wrong! The fun has only just begun. Being sat down for hours on end is sure to make your children lose their cool, more than a little bit. That's where the pre-planned games, downloaded movies, books, and entertainment come in real handy.

We'll be taking a little look at the Valsalva maneuver later on in the book, however, just as a little heads-up, children find this to be very difficult. Colds are notorious for spreading very easily when young and this only exacerbates the situation. It's essentially holding your nose and blowing but there are other options to help with those sore ears. Bring some sweets for them to suck on whilst first climbing and starting the descent. If your kids are allowed, then try chewing gum as an alternative or a pacifier if they are younger. Hydration is key here so, as always, drink some water.

Different age groups of children will respond to travelling in a multitude of ways. You'll need to try to find a path that works for you and the people around you whilst on a flight. Keep at it, use the notes pages I've hidden in the back of this book to help you remember the things that worked.

Unfortunately, for children under 2 years old, flying on a larger aeroplane can be quite intimidating and this leads to a lot of upset when onboard. There are, however, a few useful things you can do to make sure you stay sane and ensure everyone stays jet lag free. Firstly, take advantage of pre-boarding. It's a great way to get on the plane first, get settled and get everyone accustomed to the surroundings. Next, buy a separate seat; now I know most airlines will allow free travel for anyone under 2 years old, however, it's far easier and actually safer to have a separate seat and use the child safety equipment provided by the airline. Lastly, make sure to pack twice the amount of necessities, quite frankly you can never have enough.

A Pilot's Guide To Beating Jet Lag For Good

OVERCOMING THE DREADED SLEEP DEFICIT

The human body will naturally work to a daily cycle, called the circadian rhythm. This rhythm is around 25 hours long, but we shorten this every day to around 24 hours... clever huh, because now every single day we're missing out on an hour of sleep.

The circadian rhythm will affect our performance of different tasks throughout the day. It's a great way to plan your day to ensure you get the best use of your precious time. This way you'll always be on top form, whatever it is you're doing.

Jobs involving manual dexterity and visual searches will ultimately follow your body temperature which will improve throughout the day and taper off toward the end as your body cools for sleeping.

Short-term memory tasks, such as remembering names and numbers, will decline as the day goes on from an optimum amount in the morning. Sleep in the REM (rapid eye movement) cycle helps with memory consolidation and so the busier a day you've been having, learning new things, you'll need more time in REM sleep to take it all in.

Your short-term memory can hold approximately 7 +/- 2 items for 30 seconds. Go ahead and try it.

On to verbal reasoning and mental arithmetic. This is best at mid-day, so if you have interviews planned with this nonsense in it, then aim for lunchtime. That's enough of that; it brings back bad memories of countless pilot aptitude tests.

Sleep patterns can be considered in terms of points. For every hour of sleep, you'll gain two points and for every hour awake you lose one point. For example, if a person goes to sleep at 10 pm and wakes at 7 am having eight hours of sleep, after sixteen hours awake and working all of their "sleep credits" will be used and so by 11 pm they would need to go to sleep again. Jet lag is the circadian dysrhythmia which causes this cycle to go completely out of whack. Your new sleep schedule is, however, able to change by an hour every day either forward or backward as needed.

It's easier to overcome all of these problems when travelling west. As we were taught in flight training, "west is best." Not much use there because I'm still planning on going east when traveling and not going around the whole globe every time!

THE COFFEE CONUNDRUM

I'll start off this chapter by admitting that *I love coffee!* It's my favorite hot drink and something I buy every day. I have gizmos and gadgets scattered all over my house and I'm glad for them every day but especially when I'm on those 4 am flights. That being said, I would, therefore, take the things I say with a pinch of salt or at least a little brown sugar.

The half-life of caffeine is 6 hours, which is to say that after 6 hours, a cup of coffee will basically have half the effect. Believe it or not, decaf coffee still has caffeine in it, just around a quarter of the amount to begin with... unless it was bloody strong.

The tried and tested pilot trick for napping when needed is to have a coffee right before sleeping. Sounds counter-intuitive but by the time you wake up from a 20-minute nap the coffee will have kicked in and, trust me, you'll be wide awake!

Coffee, tea, and anything that contains caffeine will make you need the loo more frequently. This has its benefits in that you'll be getting up more, stretching your legs, and wandering down the cabin. It also means you'll be losing a lot of water so make sure to drink clear liquids throughout the day as well. Carbonated drinks aren't really much of a substitute here, so maybe try herbal teas if you're not keen on just water.

Coffee, as far as I can ascertain, has a load of health benefits. Amongst them is the lower risk of heart disease, lower risk of Parkinson's and Alzheimer's, improved repair, and greater general alertness. Now those are the points I've found to back up my addiction and I'm sticking to it. What can I say? I warned you I love coffee.

Now onto the downside which mainly is sleep. Obviously, if you're dosing up on caffeine late at night, you will more than likely have trouble sleeping. Just make sure to not have a drink late in the evening and you'll be fine. The rate caffeine is metabolised will depend highly on you as an individual and so the best idea is to learn from experience. If you're going to have coffee then make sure you leave enough time to get a good night's sleep before the flight.

As coffee connoisseurs all over will tell you, there are hundreds of different notes in the flavors. More, in fact, than wine has. So, I'm sure there's a flavour out there for everyone. It's a passion of mine and one which I am trying my best to keep. Each and every coffee is different. There are some great little devices that allow you to travel with easy access to decent coffee. If you're a coffee-lover, I'd recommend investing in a travel mug. More and more airport coffee shops will give you a fairly sizeable discount just for using your own cup.

THE BEST IDEAS WHEN IN YOUR SEAT

Make sure to move! Most people get comfy in their seats and simply sit down the entire flight. Not the best idea at all really, as your body aches and you'll struggle to go to sleep. This is also the reason many people can experience blood clots and the reason those strangely tight socks are sold onboard to help with this.

If you've ever given blood, you'll know all about the exercises they make you do. If you haven't then it's basically to keep the blood pumping around you while they drain you of the good red stuff. Have a quick look at those exercises online, because they are great for when you're sitting to stop your body from cramping up. Notable exercises include squeezing your fist into a ball and releasing, cletching your glutes, and moving your feet in a circular motion.

The Valsalva Maneuver. Now many of you will know of this but not know the official name. This is when you exhale moderately forcefully against a closed airway, usually pinching your nose.

In other words, you hold your nose and blow. It's used to equalise pressure between your inner ear as you ascend, or decend, and ensures that you don't burst your eardrum. Flying with a cold is a bad idea because you can easily have blocked sinuses which stop this maneuver from working. You'll then burst an eardrum fairly quickly and trust me, you'll be in a lot of pain. Having known people to do this, I'd recommend decongestants if you struggle with blocked sinuses.

I've touched upon breathing techniques previously however, I think it's worth a little mention here as well. There are so many different ones out there and they're all very easy to do whilst sitting in your seat. Have a look at Wim Hof, Pranayama, and Holotropic breathing if you're interested further. I'll expand on the 'box' breathing technique below, which I personally use regularly, to get you started;

Box breathing - Great for meditation and relaxation. Sitting upright, slowly exhale through your mouth, getting all the oxygen out of your lungs. Then inhale slowly and deeply through your nose to the count of four. Hold your breath for another count of four. Exhale to the count of four. Hold your breath to..you guessed it..the count of four. Repeat. The 4x4 technique, box breathing; not that tricky but really quite good.

Remember to drink a consistent supply of water because your whole body will be slowly drying out up there. Ever noticed how when you get off a plane your hands are dry, eyes sting, and your nose is full of crusty bits. That's not great, is it? Drink and hydrate!

UNLEASHING YOUR INNER HYPOCHONDRIAC

When I first started flying I would get all the colds and illnesses under the sun. I would go to work perfectly healthy, top-up on vitamins and try to eat well but I kept getting ill. It wasn't until I started literally applying anti-bac gel everywhere that I started to feel well after going to work. The moral of that short story is this, *always* carry anti-bacterial gel!

Your seating position on an aircraft can influence how well you feel when getting off. Sitting over the wheels in the middle of the plane is the best idea if you tend to get a bit queasy. The aircraft is most stable at this point, much like a pendulum, and so you shouldn't get too much of the lumps and bumps. Sitting at the back is the worst bet; it can get pretty interesting back there in bad turbulence. Sitting at the front is good, not only for getting out first but also for legroom and comfort. This is why it costs extra on most airlines, but I suppose you get what you pay for.

A Pilot's Guide To Beating Jet Lag For Good

The sheer amount of illness spread on an aeroplane is staggering. The worst places to find these bugs and germs are on your tray table, armrests, and obviously toilets. The armrests simply do not ever get cleaned. Make sure to wash your hands after using the toilets and use that trusted anti-bac gel at every opportunity. Personally, I start the day by whacking a load onto my hands and coating the surfaces I'm likely to touch.

Eating food onboard is interesting, to say the least. Each can, packet, and coating has been touched by at least 5 people before getting to your mouth, and who knows what they've been touching. Try to not touch the things you're eating and tentatively hold onto the corners; you'll look very odd but you can smile on the inside knowing you won't be strapped to a toilet for the rest of your holiday. Now you can always use that trusted bottle of hand-sanitiser as well if you'd like.

Air conditioning. For most out there, this will be a massive cause of debate. A lot of people will say never have that recycled air aimed anywhere toward your face and these people go on to spend most of the flight turning everyone's air conditioner off in a four-row radius. So, to explain once and for all, use the air conditioner! Its recycled air but has been passed through a "particulate arrestor" which essentially tries to rid it of impurities. It's also mixed with a load of air from the outside, via the engines. Aiming it toward your face will keep the air around you from stagnating and should help keep those germs away from you. Plus you'll be a decent temperature so that's a bonus.

If I'm to sum up this chapter in a few words, which I am about to, you will probably be able to guess what I would say. But just in case you haven't, and just in case some random person picks up this book to this exact page, remember one thing…

USE HAND SANITISER AS IF YOUR LIFE DEPENDS ON IT!

A Pilot's Guide To Beating Jet Lag For Good

THE QUICKEST WAY TO WAKE UP ALERT

As mentioned in previous chapters, your body needs REM, Deep, and Light sleep throughout the night. If you don't get enough of one type your body will make up for the deficit the next night. So if you have an early wake-up call in the morning, this will usually reduce the amount of REM sleep you will get. The next night you will get more REM sleep, missing out on light sleep in its place, and feel tired.

Light has a massive influence on how alert you will feel when you wake up. Your body and brain will get into a routine linked to the daily cycle of the sun. This routine helps you fall asleep when it gets dark and to wake up when it starts getting light. If you need to, use an eye mask to help fall asleep when it's light outside. I would recommend switching the lights on slowly when you wake up, open the curtains and get some natural light to help start the day.

As discussed in other chapters, your body is

on a constant circadian rhythm. These rhythms can be interrupted frequently and interruptions lead to poor sleep quality. The best idea is to shape your rhythms to what best suits you and your schedule. If you need to, take a few weeks and try going to bed at the same time, waking up at the same time, and eating regularly. This completely resets your sleep pattern and allows you to get into the routine your body craves. It's hard on shift work to do this but worth it in the long run.

Stress is an interesting topic. The sheer amount of negative effects it can have on your body is mind-boggling. I personally believe that long exposure to stress will take years off your life. To limit stress as much as possible I take the time out from my daily routine to relax and release the tension. Take 5 minutes before bed to evaluate the day and to unwind; trust me, you'll feel the benefits.

This little trick will apply when you're flying and also at home. If you ensure that you have a glass of water by your side and upon first waking up, make sure to sit up and have a large sip. The process of sitting up will make you feel more awake and the water will start your body's natural process in breaking its fast for the night. If it's ice cold water, even better, it can have some really good health benefits, it greatly increases your body's metabolism for the day and improves oxygen flow as well.

FOOD AND HEALTH TIPS

This chapter is essentially about healthy eating. The number of calories you need to take in depends on you as an individual. Which body type you are? There are three types; ectomorph, mesomorph, and endomorph. It's worth having a look online to see which category you fall under in more detail but I've listed the basics below;

An ectomorph is usually lean and long, has trouble gaining muscle. A mesomorph will be larger, pear-shaped body and often stores body fat. An endomorph will be muscular and well-built, with a high metabolism and responsive muscle cells.

How much do you exercise? Most people aim for around 10,000 steps per day. The list goes on.

Food is a huge part of travelling for everyone and when you're up in the air with very limited options, you have to know what to eat. I recommend seeing the package to look at the sheer amount of oddities that go into your food on-board and then make your decision.

When alcohol is in the bloodstream, it interferes with the absorption of oxygen in the blood. Higher altitudes have less oxygen in the air to begin with and so the effect is magnified, and you end up getting less oxygen to the brain. Other people might be complete drunks at all elevations.

The aircraft you fly commercially will always be pressurised, usually to around 8000ft. equivalent pressure. This is around the same as climbing Mount Taranaki in New Zealand. It's harder for your blood to pump oxygen around your body and can make you a little light-headed with alcohol. If it weren't pressurised, however, at 36000ft. you'd have around 45 seconds before you passed out from hypoxia. Not a pleasant thought.

Now foods to avoid. I'll give you a list: Salty snacks, beans, cruciferous vegetables, fried foods, spicy foods, carbonated drinks, and alcohol. The main reason for avoiding these foods is gas. High fiber content and sodium levels can cause gas which is not a pleasant experience when influenced by altitude. Try to avoid these foods the day before but at the very least for a few hours before flying to avoid that stomach lurch in the air.

Good foods: Lean protein, oranges, bananas, yoghurt, nuts, herbal teas, and most importantly water. Fruits are always a good idea but oranges and bananas are just great. The oranges provide vitamin C to help fight all these nasty germs I'm talking about and the bananas provide potassium which stops cramps. Obviously, always drink a lot of water; it's never a good idea to be dehydrated at the best of times.

Ginger root is a great supplement to the diet. It's nice with some hot water and a slice of lemon. It helps to relieve the tension and to calm your body. Try having a glass before bed and see if you feel any benefits. I have a glass now and again to aid sleep and also to settle the stomach after having a few dodgy crew foods.

HIGHLY EFFECTIVE HABITS

Habits are a great idea to get into the routine before you travel. Use these habits as guidelines and get into the regular pattern before going on a flight. Try to get necessities ready the night before. Put the trusty hand sanitiser in with your toiletries in a clear bag for easy access. Get down the travel pillows from the attic and most importantly, get all the chargers you need for the gadgets. Being prepared for the day limits the amount of stress you'll be under while queueing at security for seemingly hours.

Security gates are an absolute nightmare for all of us, including crew. The things seem to beep and buzz of their own accord. The thing to do is arrive that little bit earlier. Get the bags sorted with electrical items on top so you can reach them. Place your passport in a side pocket if possible and have your boarding pass ready on your mobile device or printed. Every little bit helps until you're the other side.

Update the time on your watch sooner rather

A Pilot's Guide To Beating Jet Lag For Good

than later. It's always worth doing this while at the airport to get accustomed to the time difference. It gives you a great way to know when to eat and helps plan the day ahead. This approach is especially useful on a long flight. I usually do it when I'm checked in and waiting for the departure board to flick over.

Seat selection. An important factor to think about. Most short-haul airlines charge for the pleasure, but usually, on long-haul, you will get a choice. It's an important one. Personally, I go for the window seats. I like looking out the window at the views, but mainly I like somewhere to rest my head. The side of the aircraft works great with a flight pillow resting on it and helps a little to get to sleep.

Before you leave the house for your flight, try to have a multi-vitamin. I've personally found that this seems to keep me on top health throughout the coming days. It could be a placebo but I'm sure that keeping all the vital minerals and vitamins up can't be a bad thing. You'll be needing all the help you can get defending your body against those weird and wonderful germs that spread so easily on aeroplanes.

Lastly, pack toiletries. It's great to have a toothbrush with you and a washcloth. They both help you to feel refreshed and ready to exit the plane. There's nothing worse than morning breath, which is ten times worse when sleeping on a plane. Plane breath. Minty fresh is a better option.

MY STRUGGLE AS A COMMERCIAL PILOT

Flying aircraft commercially for a living is a completely different ballgame when it comes to being jet lagged and fatigued. As an airline pilot, you need to get used to jumping between time zones on a very regular basis and making sure your health doesn't suffer too much along the way.

I've touched upon the information I've gleaned along my travels and hopefully, you'll now be able to avoid the pitfalls I most definitely fell for early on in my career. Trust me; it's a thin line between being tired and being fatigued. The latter *will* kill you in the long run.

I can remember coming back from a long flight and being horrendously tired. I managed to get some sleep at 7 am, after what turned into a 22-hour day with the delays, where I slept for about 4 hours. Not much at all to recover. I thought I'd head to the gym and go for a swim to try to rejuvenate my poor body. After showering I changed into my clothes and genuinely forgot if I'd showered, as I'd

A Pilot's Guide To Beating Jet Lag For Good

have been wet from the pool either way. I showered again. Jet lag has a huge impact on short-term memory and over long periods, it will affect long-term memory as well. It really is awful.

I've mentioned hand sanitiser a lot in this book and I don't want to bore you with it again. What I will ask you to do is try something next time you go on a flight; wash your hands in a proper sink when you're on the ground right after you get off the plane. Honestly, no matter how hard you try, your hand will be full of filth. I've tried washing my hands in the sink onboard right before I get off and yet still when I get on the ground the water doesn't look too pretty. It's amazing. Gray water flows off your hands every time!

Coffee has been a massive influence in my career and I am forever grateful for it. Ground-school and all the exams you have to take if you want to become a commercial pilot are very intensive and you'll need a good bit of caffeine to help out with those long nights of study. A little word of warning though and to speak with some experience in the issue, I'll let your imaginations make up the rest. Don't have too many energy drinks before a flight. It's a tight squeeze back there in your seat and even tighter in the cockpit. Those Imodium will come in handy if your stomach isn't up to the job. Not a nice experience and honestly makes you wish you had some windows, even at 36000ft.

Being a commercial pilot has been an absolute privilege in my life. I've had plenty of tough times, not only throughout training but also in my career. That being said, it has always been a career that I have enjoyed and hope to enjoy for a long time to come. Serious fatigue and tiredness will always be a major concern with both short-haul and long-haul airlines in shift work patterns. It's only really becoming apparent over the last decade or so, just how detrimental it is to your health to operate in such a way. I use as many ways as I can think of to eliminate the risk of tiredness and if needs be, I may not come into work at all if I am fatigued.

I hope that everyone can experience the absolute joys of aviation and stay healthy whilst doing so. There are so many wonderful places to visit and fantastic things to see. Have fun!

A Pilot's Guide To Beating Jet Lag For Good

THE ONLY WAY IS UP!

Well that's it; the last chapter is here. For those who have stuck it out, well done! For those who haven't, well enjoy getting ill on your precious holiday.

There are many ways and means to help protect yourself and your general well-being while travelling this rather blue looking planet. I have covered a few but not all. Feel free to adapt, change, and rethink my suggestions. These are guidelines to follow to ensure the struggle, we all face while on our adventures, isn't too difficult.

Hopefully, you'll have gained a few more insights into how to avoid jet lag once and for all. These tips and tricks should keep you in good stead for the future and allow you to get to your destination feeling well-rested, happy, and--most of all--healthy.

Make sure to enjoy all the travels and adventures you go on. There are simply just so many opportunities out there and it really would be a shame to miss them. Take your children or partner, take a camera, and take a good book. You'll be amazed at how adaptable the body is; and how even though you've just crossed countless time zones in one sitting, you can still bounce back and have a great holiday.

Flying is an art, not just for the pilots and crew but for the passengers as well. Trying to survive on a long-haul flight is an effort. Trust me. I've been there. Short-haul can have its own challenges. That's for sure. It's also a massive privilege. Being able, as humans, to fly has given humanity so much. Ensuring we stay healthy while doing it is the least we can do.

Good luck everyone and I hope you go on to share insights with your friends and family. The only way is up!

A Pilot's Guide To Beating Jet Lag For Good

Top 10 Points to Remember!

1. Use hand sanitiser on absolutely everything humanly possible

2. Well timed sleep is crutial to feeling healthy

3. Drink plenty of water throughout the day

4. Good earplugs are a solid investment

5. Pack some imodium, before you find out the hard way

6. The air conditioning onboard is there to be used

7. Drink caffeine wisely

8. Gadgets help with so much, bring them and a charger

9. Pack a toothbrush to avoid that gnarly breath

10. Have fun, relax, and enjoy your travels!

WHAT DID YOU THINK?

First of all, thank you for purchasing this book, A Pilot's Guide to Beating Jet Lag for Good. I know you could have picked any number of books to read, there are so many good ones out there. Though, not enough on the topic of jet lag I must admit. I am extremely grateful that you picked this one.

I hope that it added some value and quality every time you travel. If so, it would be really nice if you could share this book with your friends and family.

I've included a link on the next page to quickly get to my Instagram profile. It's a great way to stay up to date and also has a lot of amazing aviation-related photos, so make sure to follow.

If you enjoyed this book and found some benefit in reading this, I'd like to hear from you and hope that you could take just a little bit of time to post a review on Amazon. Your feedback and support will really help to improve future projects and make this book even better.

With your help and support there will likely be more books to follow in the edition of 'A Pilot's Guide to..'

I truly wish you all the best for your travels and for your future success.

S Price

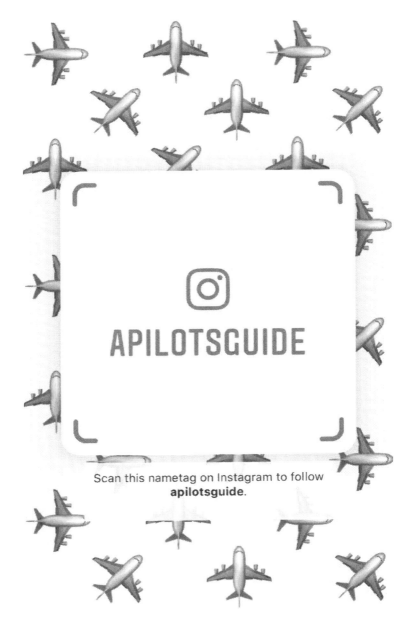

Scan this nametag on Instagram to follow **apilotsguide**.

A Pilot's Guide To Beating Jet Lag For Good

NOTES

Use these pages as you wish. Add your own notes and keep track of your travels and how you feel. I find it useful to log my flights and how I felt afterward, seeing if I get ill or need more sleep and things I can change next time to stop it from happening.

S Price

-
-
-

A Pilot's Guide To Beating Jet Lag For Good

-

-

-

Printed in Great Britain
by Amazon